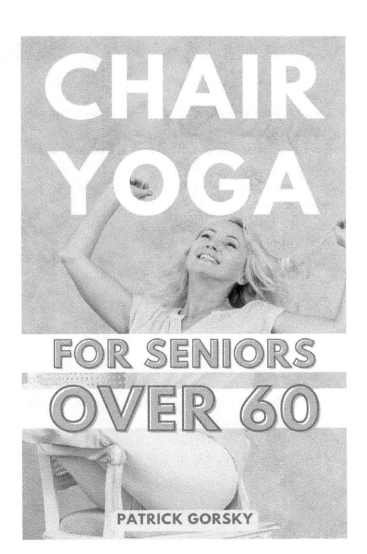

CHAIR YOGA

FOR SENIORS
OVER 60

PATRICK GORSKY

The "Chair Yoga for Seniors over 60" is an invaluable resource. It delivers a holistic approach to yoga, tailored to the unique needs of older adults, enhancing flexibility and overall health. With its user-friendly instructions and a wide range of exercises, it makes yoga accessible and enjoyable for seniors, promoting well-being in a comfortable and supportive manner. This guide is a must-have for anyone looking to stay active and vibrant in their golden years.

JOHN P., SCOTTSBLUFF, NEBRASKA

This tutorial offers a comprehensive yoga program designed with older adults in mind, promoting flexibility, balance, and relaxation. Its step-by-step instructions and variety of exercises make yoga easily accessible to seniors, fostering well-being and vitality in a gentle and supportive way. This guide is a fantastic tool for seniors seeking to enhance their overall health and quality of life.

FELIX K., MIKKELI, FINLAND

Thanks for it. This is a remarkable resource that empowers older adults to embrace yoga, enhancing their flexibility and inner peace through expertly designed exercises. It's an indispensable companion for seniors on their journey to improved well-being.

ALICE P., JUNDAH, QUEENSLAND

Patrick Gorsky

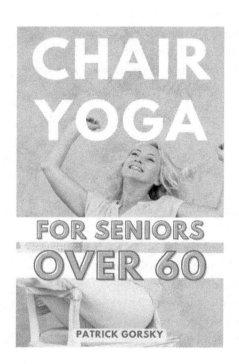

For Noah

In moments of joy, your understanding
shines brightly. I want to express my
appreciation, dear friend, for your unwavering
and consistent support.

For Nyomi

Grateful for a time of rejuvenation and
bliss, Together we climbed, our spirits entwined.
I offer my gratitude, dear friends, for the
cherished memory's comforting embrace.

PREFACE

A GOLDEN PATH TO VITALITY AND SERENITY IN YOUR GOLDEN YEARS

In a world that never stops moving, where the pace of life seems to quicken with each passing day, we find ourselves racing through the years, often neglecting the very vessels that have carried us through life's countless journeys – our bodies. In our quest to keep up with the relentless demands of modern life, we sometimes forget to pause, breathe, and care for ourselves.

But as the years accumulate and the calendar pages turn, there comes a time when our bodies begin to whisper their needs more persistently, reminding us that it's never too late to prioritize our well-being. This book, "Chair Yoga for Seniors Over 60," is an invitation to embark on a remarkable journey of self-discovery, renewal, and transformation.

As we navigate the golden years, life presents us with a unique set of challenges and opportunities. The joints may creak, and the muscles may tighten, but our spirits remain as vibrant and youthful as ever. Aging, after all, is a privilege denied to many, and it is within our grasp to make these years not only meaningful but truly enjoyable.

Yoga, a practice that has been cultivated and revered for centuries, holds the key to unlocking a world of vitality, serenity, and strength – regardless of age or physical condition. Chair yoga, an adaptation of the traditional yoga practice, has emerged as a gentle yet powerful tool for nurturing the body, mind, and soul, particularly for those in their senior years.

This book is a heartfelt testament to the power of chair yoga in rejuvenating your life, improving your overall well-being, and embracing the fullness of your senior years with grace and enthusiasm. It is a roadmap to a healthier, happier, and more harmonious existence.

Within these pages, you will discover a treasure trove of wisdom, practical guidance, and inspiring stories that demonstrate the remarkable benefits of chair yoga for seniors over 60. Each chapter is designed to be a stepping stone on your journey to improved flexibility, balance, strength, and inner peace.

As you delve into these pages, you will encounter a diverse range of chair yoga poses and sequences tailored to address the specific needs and challenges of seniors. From gentle stretches to soothing breathing exercises, you will find a wealth of practices that will empower you to reconnect with your body and embrace the joy of movement.

But this book offers more than just physical exercises. It delves into the heart of yoga philosophy, helping you cultivate mindfulness, resilience, and a deeper understanding of the mind-body connection. As you read, you will explore the ancient principles of yoga and how they can be seamlessly integrated into your daily life, enriching your existence in ways you may never have imagined.

Furthermore, "Chair Yoga for Seniors Over 60" places a strong emphasis on the importance of community and emotional well-being. You will encounter heartfelt stories from individuals who have embarked on their own chair yoga journeys and have experienced profound transformations in their lives. These personal narratives serve as beacons of hope, reminding us that it is never too late to embark on a path of self-discovery and renewal.

In our fast-paced world, it's easy to forget the importance of self-care, especially as we age. Yet, this book is a testament to the fact that self-care knows no age limits. It is an act of love, respect, and gratitude toward the body that has carried us through a lifetime of experiences.

So, my dear reader, I urge you to embrace this book as a trusted companion on your journey to a more vibrant and fulfilling life.

Let its pages inspire you, its practices rejuvenate you, and its stories uplift you. As you embark on this path of self-discovery through chair yoga, may you find a renewed sense of purpose, vitality, and joy in every moment of your senior years.

May this book be a source of light and guidance, reminding you that the golden years are not a time of decline but an opportunity for growth, transformation, and the unwavering pursuit of well-being. Embrace the wisdom within these pages, and let the journey of chair yoga lead you to a life filled with grace, strength, and enduring joy.

With open hearts and open minds, let us embark on this empowering journey together, one breath, one pose, one page at a time.

Patrick Gorsky

TABLE OF CONTENTS

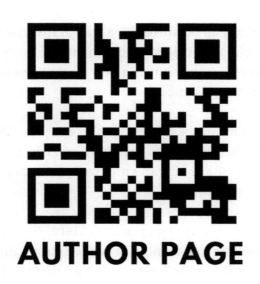

AUTHOR PAGE

ENTRY

Welcome to the world of Chair Yoga, a transformative and uplifting practice specially designed to enhance the lives of seniors over 60. In the pages of this book, we embark on a journey that will not only introduce you to the wonderful world of Chair Yoga but also inspire you to embrace this empowering practice wholeheartedly.

Life beyond 60 is a time of wisdom, grace, and, most importantly, an opportunity for self-care and personal growth. In this chapter, we explore the unique challenges and joys that come with aging and why Chair Yoga is the perfect tool for seniors to navigate this phase of life. Let's break free from stereotypes and embrace the limitless potential within.

Yoga is more than just physical postures; it's a way of life that harmonizes mind, body, and spirit. In this chapter, we delve into the rich history and philosophy of yoga, demystifying its essence and showing how Chair Yoga can be a gateway to a more mindful and balanced existence.

Learn why the chair is your new best friend in this chapter. We explore how this simple piece of furniture becomes your yoga mat, offering stability, support, and accessibility. Discover how the chair can empower you to access yoga's benefits, regardless of your physical abilities.

Breathing is the foundation of any yoga practice. Here, we explore the art of mindful breathing, unlocking its potential to reduce stress, improve lung capacity, and boost energy levels. With Chair Yoga, you'll find that the breath is your guiding force towards serenity.

Chair Yoga isn't about contorting your body into impossible shapes. It's about gentle movements that promote flexibility, strength, and balance. Discover how these accessible poses can alleviate common aches and pains, enhance mobility, and foster a sense of empowerment.

Mindfulness is the key to a peaceful and joyful life. In this chapter, we delve into the practice of mindfulness and how it intertwines with Chair Yoga. Learn how to stay present, release worries, and cultivate a positive outlook on life.

Mental health is as important as physical health. Here, we explore the mind-body connection and how Chair Yoga can promote mental clarity, reduce anxiety, and enhance emotional well-being. Discover how you can create a sanctuary of peace within yourself.

Chair Yoga isn't just for your mat; it's a way of life. This chapter offers practical tips on incorporating Chair Yoga into your daily routine. Whether you're at home, in the office, or on a journey, you'll find ways to stay committed to your practice.

Yoga is a journey best taken with others. In this chapter, we explore the importance of community in your yoga practice. Discover how connecting with like-minded individuals can enhance your experience and provide a sense of belonging.

Aging doesn't mean the end of growth; it's an opportunity for lifelong learning. We conclude our journey by encouraging you to keep exploring, experimenting, and evolving your Chair Yoga practice. Your golden years are a canvas, and Chair Yoga is your brush.

As we close the final chapter of this book, I hope you are inspired to delve deeper into the world of Chair Yoga for seniors over 60. This practice has the power to uplift your spirit, enhance your well-being, and lead you toward a life filled with joy, vitality, and purpose. Your journey has just begun, and the chair is your trusty companion on this path to self-discovery and empowerment. So, take a seat, breathe, and let Chair Yoga transform your life in ways you never imagined. The best is yet to come!

CHAPTER 1
Seated Mountain Pose

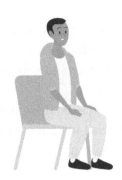

In the world of Chair Yoga, the Seated Mountain Pose stands tall as the foundational posture, much like the majestic mountains that inspire its name. This seemingly simple yet deeply powerful pose serves as the cornerstone upon which your Chair Yoga practice is built. In this chapter, we will explore the Seated Mountain Pose, its benefits, variations, and the profound impact it can have on your physical and mental well-being.

Seated Mountain Pose Unveiled

At first glance, Seated Mountain Pose may appear as just sitting up straight in a chair. However, when practiced mindfully, it embodies the essence of balance, stability, and strength. To perform the Seated Mountain Pose:

1. Begin by sitting tall in your chair with your feet flat on the ground, hip-width apart.

2. Ensure your spine is straight, and your shoulders are relaxed.

3. Place your hands gently on your thighs, palms facing downward, or rest them on your lap with your palms facing upward to receive energy.

4. Close your eyes or maintain a soft gaze forward.

5. Take a moment to focus on your breath. Inhale deeply through your nose, allowing your chest to rise, and exhale slowly through your mouth, letting go of any tension.

6. Feel the connection between your sit bones and the chair, grounding you like the roots of a mountain.

The Benefits of Seated Mountain Pose

1. Posture Improvement: Seated Mountain Pose is a powerful tool for correcting poor posture, which can be a common issue in our sedentary lifestyles. Regular practice strengthens the back muscles, encouraging you to sit and stand with a more aligned spine.

2. Stress Reduction: As you sit in stillness, focusing on your breath, you cultivate mindfulness. This reduces stress and promotes a sense of calm, which is invaluable in our busy lives.

3. Improved Circulation: Sitting tall in Seated Mountain Pose opens up the chest, facilitating better lung function and blood circulation. This can be especially beneficial for those with respiratory issues or circulation problems.

4. Increased Awareness: This foundational pose brings attention to the present moment. As you become aware of your body's alignment and sensations, you develop a deeper connection with yourself.

5. Mind-Body Harmony: Seated Mountain Pose bridges the gap between the physical and mental aspects of yoga. It serves as a conduit for aligning your body, mind, and spirit, promoting holistic well-being.

Variations and Adaptations

One of the beauty of Chair Yoga is its adaptability. Seated Mountain Pose can be customized to suit your unique needs and abilities:

1. Dynamic Seated Mountain: Incorporate gentle movements by swaying side to side or rotating your torso. This adds a dynamic element to the pose, increasing flexibility and range of motion.

2. Breathing Focus: Emphasize deep breathing in Seated Mountain Pose by inhaling deeply, raising your arms overhead, and exhaling as you lower them. This enhances lung capacity and relaxation.

3. Using Props: For those with limited mobility or balance issues, consider using props like yoga blocks or a cushion to support your practice.

This can help you sit comfortably while maintaining the essence of the pose.

Closing Thoughts

Seated Mountain Pose is not just an exercise; it's a state of being. It reminds us to stand strong, rooted like a mountain, and to weather life's storms with grace and resilience.

As you delve into the heart of Chair Yoga, return to Seated Mountain Pose often. Let it be your refuge, your reset button, and your guide as you explore the vast landscape of this transformative practice. From this stable foundation, you will embark on a journey that leads to greater self-discovery, health, and a renewed sense of vitality. Seated Mountain Pose is your gateway to a life lived in balance, just like the mountains that inspire it.

CHAPTER 2
Seated Forward Bend

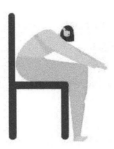

Within the gentle embrace of a chair, the Seated Forward Bend pose blossoms as a sanctuary of serenity in the realm of Chair Yoga. This rejuvenating posture holds the potential to transform your practice and your well-being. In this chapter, we will explore the Seated Forward Bend in depth, unraveling its many benefits, variations, and the profound peace it can bring to your body, mind, and spirit.

The Seated Forward Bend Unveiled

Seated Forward Bend, often referred to as "Paschimottanasana" in traditional yoga, is a restorative pose that offers a myriad of physical and mental benefits. In Chair Yoga, it is adapted for seated practice, making it accessible to people of all ages and abilities.

To perform Seated Forward Bend in a chair:

1. Begin by sitting tall in your chair, with your feet flat on the ground, hip-width apart.

2. Place your hands on your thighs, palms facing downward, or rest them on your lap, palms facing upward.

3. Inhale deeply, elongating your spine, and exhale slowly, allowing your shoulders to relax.

4. As you inhale, lift your arms overhead, lengthening your spine even further.

5. Exhale and hinge at your hips, gently leaning forward while keeping your back straight.

6. Allow your hands to reach toward your feet, ankles, or shins, depending on your flexibility.

7. Hold this position for a few breaths, feeling a gentle stretch along your spine and the back of your legs.

8. To release, inhale and slowly return to an upright position, keeping your spine long.

The Benefits of Seated Forward Bend

1. Spinal Flexibility: Seated Forward Bend is a gentle way to stretch and maintain the flexibility of your spine, which can diminish with age. This can alleviate back pain and improve posture.

2. Stress Reduction: The forward bend position encourages deep relaxation. As you surrender to gravity, you release tension and reduce stress, promoting mental clarity and calm.

3. Digestive Health: This pose gently massages your abdominal organs, aiding in digestion and relieving discomfort associated with gastrointestinal issues.

4. Improved Posture: Seated Forward Bend promotes awareness of your spinal alignment. Over time, this awareness can extend to your everyday posture, helping you sit and stand with better posture.

5. Mind-Body Connection: As you fold forward, you're encouraged to turn inward, fostering mindfulness and introspection.

Variations and Adaptations

In Chair Yoga, Seated Forward Bend offers an array of variations and adaptations to cater to your unique needs:

1. Supported Forward Bend: Place a cushion or yoga block on your lap and gently lean forward, resting your forehead on the support. This variation provides extra comfort and encourages deeper relaxation.

2. One-Legged Forward Bend: Lift one leg off the ground and extend it forward, hinging at the hip to reach for your toes or shin. This variation emphasizes hamstring flexibility.

3. Twisting Forward Bend: Incorporate a gentle twist by reaching one hand across your body and placing it on the opposite knee. As you fold forward, allow the twist to deepen the stretch in your spine.

4. Chair-Assisted Forward Bend: Hold onto the sides of your chair as you fold forward for added stability, especially if balance is a concern.

Closing Thoughts

Seated Forward Bend in Chair Yoga invites you to surrender to the present moment, finding solace in the simplicity of the pose. It is a gentle reminder that even in the hustle and bustle of life, there exists a tranquil space within, waiting to be explored and cherished. Through this practice, you will discover a deep sense of self-awareness, peace, and rejuvenation. Allow the Seated Forward Bend to be your gateway to serenity and a steadfast companion on your journey to holistic well-being. In the gentle curve of your body as you lean forward, you will find the profound arc of tranquility that Chair Yoga offers.

CHAPTER 3
Seated Cat-Cow Stretch

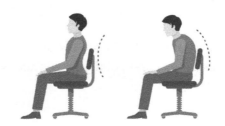

The Seated Cat-Cow Stretch, a dynamic and invigorating pose, transcends the boundaries of traditional yoga and flourishes as a vital practice within Chair Yoga. This chapter unveils the profound benefits, variations, and transformative potential that Seated Cat-Cow Stretch brings to your physical and emotional well-being. Within the gentle curvature of your spine, lies a world of rejuvenation and inner harmony waiting to be explored.

The Seated Cat-Cow Stretch Unveiled

The Seated Cat-Cow Stretch is an adaptation of the traditional Cat-Cow Stretch, designed for seated practice in a chair. It combines fluid movement and conscious breathing to enhance the flexibility and vitality of your spine, even while seated.

To perform Seated Cat-Cow Stretch in a chair:

1. Begin by sitting tall in your chair with your feet flat on the ground, hip-width apart.

2. Place your hands on your thighs, palms facing downward, or rest them on your lap, palms facing upward.

3. Inhale deeply, arching your back and lifting your chest toward the sky. Allow your shoulders to roll back and your gaze to lift slightly.

4. Exhale slowly, rounding your back like a cat, tucking your chin to your chest, and drawing your navel toward your spine.

5. Continue to flow between these two movements, inhaling as you transition into the Cow position (arched back) and exhaling as you transition into the Cat position (rounded back).

6. Repeat this sequence for several breaths, moving with intention and fluidity.

The Benefits of Seated Cat-Cow Stretch

1. Spinal Health: Seated Cat-Cow Stretch is a gift to your spine. It encourages flexibility and maintains the natural curvature of your vertebral column. This can help alleviate back pain and improve posture.

2. Enhanced Circulation: As you alternate between the two positions, you stimulate blood flow to the spine, enhancing its overall health and functionality.

3. Stress Reduction: The synchronized movement with breath cultivates mindfulness and relaxation. It can be a powerful tool for reducing stress and promoting mental clarity.

4. Digestive Health: The gentle compression and release of the abdominal organs in this stretch can aid digestion and alleviate discomfort related to digestive issues.

5. Emotional Release: Seated Cat-Cow Stretch provides an avenue for releasing emotional tension and promoting a sense of well-being. The rhythmic movement can have a calming and grounding effect on your mind.

Variations and Adaptations

Chair Yoga thrives on adaptability, and Seated Cat-Cow Stretch offers a range of variations to suit your unique needs:

1. Gentle Cat-Cow: If you have limited mobility or find the traditional movement challenging, simplify it by moving just your shoulders and upper back. Imagine creating a wave-like motion through your upper spine.

2. Cat-Cow with Breath Emphasis: Focus on the breath aspect of this stretch by elongating your inhalations and exhalations. This deepens your connection with your breath and enhances relaxation.

3. Seated Cat-Cow with Twist: Combine the Cat-Cow Stretch with a gentle twist. Inhale in the Cow position, and as you exhale, twist to one side, bringing one hand to the backrest of your chair. Inhale back to the center and exhale to the other side.

Closing Thoughts

Seated Cat-Cow Stretch in Chair Yoga serves as a testament to the adaptability and transformative power of this practice. As you flow through these graceful movements, you reconnect with the fluidity of life itself. The curvature of your spine mirrors the natural ebb and flow of existence, inviting you to embrace change with grace and resilience. Through this practice, you not only nurture the health of your spine but also cultivate a deeper connection with your inner self. Let Seated Cat-Cow Stretch be your guide to nurturing both your physical and spiritual well-being, as you embrace the vitality that Chair Yoga offers. In the arch and round of your spine, you'll find the gentle dance of transformation and healing, inviting you to explore the profound depths of this transformative practice.

CHAPTER 4

Seated Twist

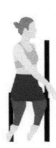

Within the realm of Chair Yoga, the Seated Twist unfurls as a potent elixir, nurturing both the physical and mental aspects of your being. In this chapter, we embark on a journey to unravel the profound benefits, versatile variations, and the transformative power that Seated Twist brings to your practice. This simple yet powerful posture is a gateway to enhanced mobility, inner harmony, and rejuvenation.

The Seated Twist Explored

The Seated Twist is a gentle yet revitalizing pose that targets your spine's flexibility and encourages a sense of balance within. It can be performed with grace and ease from the comfort of your chair.

To practice Seated Twist in a chair:

1. Begin by sitting tall in your chair with your feet flat on the ground, hip-width apart.

2. Place your hands on your thighs, palms facing downward, or rest them on your lap, palms facing upward.

3. Inhale deeply, elongating your spine, and exhale slowly, allowing your shoulders to relax.

4. On an inhale, gently twist your upper body to one side, turning from your waist and keeping your hips rooted to the chair.

5. As you exhale, maintain the twist, and deepen it slightly if comfortable, using your opposite hand to hold onto the backrest of the chair.

6. Keep your spine long and your gaze soft.

7. Breathe steadily in this twist for several breaths, allowing the gentle rotation to create space in your spine and awaken your inner vitality.

8. To release, inhale, and slowly return to the center, and then repeat on the other side.

The Benefits of Seated Twist

1. Spinal Health: Seated Twist promotes spinal health by enhancing its flexibility. Regular practice can alleviate back pain and improve overall posture.

2. Digestive Wellness: The gentle compression and release of your abdominal organs during the twist stimulate digestion and alleviate discomfort related to digestive issues.

3. Detoxification: The twisting motion encourages the flushing of toxins from your body, promoting detoxification and revitalization.

4. Mental Clarity: Seated Twist fosters a sense of balance and inner harmony. As you release tension in your spine, you may also find mental clarity and emotional equilibrium.

5. Enhanced Mobility: This pose gently stretches and lubricates your spine, enhancing mobility and range of motion, which can be particularly beneficial for those with limited mobility.

Variations and Adaptations

Seated Twist in Chair Yoga offers a spectrum of variations to cater to your unique needs:

1. Supported Seated Twist: If you have balance concerns or require extra support, hold onto the sides of your chair or use a cushion to sit on for added height and stability.

2. Half-Seated Twist: If the full twist is challenging, begin by practicing a half-twist, turning your upper body to one side and keeping the opposite hand on your thigh for support.

3. Seated Twist with a Forward Fold: Combine Seated Twist with a forward fold by hinging at the hips and reaching for your foot or ankle on the same side as your twist. This variation intensifies the stretch.

4. Dynamic Seated Twist: Incorporate dynamic movement by moving in and out of the twist with your breath, enhancing the fluidity of the practice.

Closing Thoughts

Seated Twist in Chair Yoga embodies the essence of adaptability, balance, and rejuvenation. It serves as a reminder that even in stillness, life continues to unfold and evolve. The gentle rotation of your spine reflects the ever-changing nature of existence, encouraging you to embrace transformation with grace and openness. Through this practice, you not only nurture the physical health of your spine but also cultivate a deeper connection with your inner self. Let Seated Twist be your compass, guiding you toward improved mobility, inner harmony, and a sense of well-being. In the spiraling motion of your body, you'll discover the profound dance of vitality and healing that Chair Yoga offers. As you explore this transformative practice, may your journey be guided by the gentle spiral of growth, renewal, and self-discovery that Seated Twist embodies.

CHAPTER 5
Seated Warrior I

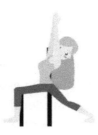

In the world of Chair Yoga, Seated Warrior I emerges as a beacon of strength and serenity. This chapter delves deep into the practice, exploring the profound benefits, adaptable variations, and the transformative potential that Seated Warrior I offers. This empowering posture, inspired by the courage and valor of a warrior, is an invitation to harness your inner strength while maintaining tranquility.

The Seated Warrior I Unveiled

Seated Warrior I is an embodiment of resilience, strength, and balance within the chair yoga practice. It allows you to tap into the essence of the traditional Warrior I pose while seated comfortably.

To practice Seated Warrior I in a chair:

1. Begin by sitting tall in your chair with your feet flat on the ground, hip-width apart.

2. Place your hands on your thighs, palms facing downward, or rest them on your lap, palms facing upward.

3. Inhale deeply, elongating your spine, and exhale slowly, allowing your shoulders to relax.

4. On an inhale, extend one leg forward, keeping your foot flat on the ground. This represents your warrior stance.

5. As you exhale, bend the opposite knee, bringing it up toward your chest. This represents your warrior's raised knee.

6. Maintain a strong and steady gaze forward, maintaining your balance.

7. Lift your arms overhead, extending them upward with your palms facing each other or touching.

8. Hold this position for several breaths, feeling the strength and stability it brings.

9. To release, exhale and slowly lower your arms and the raised knee, returning to the starting position.

10. Repeat the pose on the other side, maintaining balance between both sides of your body.

The Benefits of Seated Warrior I

1. Strength and Stability: Seated Warrior I builds strength in the legs, shoulders, and core muscles, which is essential for maintaining stability and balance in everyday activities.

2. Improved Posture: This pose encourages an upright and confident posture, enhancing your overall body alignment.

3. Mental Focus: Seated Warrior I requires concentration to maintain balance, fostering mental clarity and mindfulness.

4. Inner Strength: As you embody the spirit of a warrior, you cultivate inner strength, resilience, and courage.

5. Flexibility: The extended leg in this pose provides a gentle stretch to the hamstrings and calf muscles, promoting flexibility.

Variations and Adaptations

Chair Yoga thrives on adaptability, and Seated Warrior I offers several variations to cater to your unique needs:

1. Supported Seated Warrior I: Hold onto the sides of your chair for added support, especially if balance is a concern.

2. Half Seated Warrior I: Practice the pose with one foot extended forward while the other remains on the ground if the full posture is challenging.

3. Dynamic Seated Warrior I: Incorporate dynamic movements by moving in and out of the pose with your breath, enhancing the flow and strength-building aspect of the practice.

4. Warrior I with Breath Emphasis: Focus on deep, intentional breaths to connect with the warrior's spirit within you.

Closing Thoughts

Seated Warrior I in Chair Yoga serves as a reminder that strength and serenity can coexist. It embodies the balance between the power of a warrior and the calm of a sage, teaching you that inner strength is cultivated not by force but by grace. Through this practice, you nurture the physical health of your body while connecting with your inner warrior, poised and unwavering in the face of life's challenges. Let Seated Warrior I be your guide to harnessing your inner strength, cultivating resilience, and finding serenity amid life's trials. In the poised stance of your body, you'll discover the profound dance of strength and tranquility that Chair Yoga offers. May your journey be guided by the warrior's spirit within, inspiring you to face each day with courage, grace, and a heart full of serenity.

CHAPTER 6
Seated Warrior II

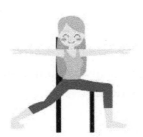

Seated Warrior II is a captivating and empowering pose in the world of Chair Yoga. This chapter will take you on an exploration of Seated Warrior II, revealing its transformative benefits, versatile adaptations, and the profound sense of power and grace it can awaken within your practice. As you engage with this dynamic posture, you'll find that the spirit of a warrior can thrive even while seated.

The Seated Warrior II Unveiled

Seated Warrior II is a reflection of both strength and grace, embodying the essence of the traditional Warrior II pose while adapted for chair practice. This pose invites you to find power and poise in the midst of stillness.

To practice Seated Warrior II in a chair:

1. Begin by sitting tall in your chair, with your feet flat on the ground and hip-width apart.

2. Place your hands on your thighs, palms facing downward, or rest them on your lap with palms facing upward.

3. Inhale deeply, elongating your spine, and exhale slowly, relaxing your shoulders.

4. On an inhale, extend one leg forward and keep the foot flat on the ground. This represents your warrior stance.

5. As you exhale, bend the opposite knee, bringing it up toward your chest, then open it to the side, mirroring the traditional Warrior II stance.

6. Keep your gaze forward, with your arms extended straight out to the sides, reaching actively in both directions.

7. Hold this posture for several breaths, feeling the strength, balance, and determination it invokes.

8. To release, exhale and slowly lower your arms and the raised knee, returning to the starting position.

9. Repeat the pose on the other side, maintaining balance between both sides of your body.

The Benefits of Seated Warrior II

1. Strength and Endurance: Seated Warrior II builds strength in the legs, shoulders, and core muscles, promoting stability and endurance.

2. Improved Posture: This pose encourages an upright and confident posture, enhancing overall body alignment.

3. Mental Focus: The need for concentration in Seated Warrior II promotes mental clarity and mindfulness.

4. Inner Empowerment: As you embody the spirit of a warrior, you cultivate inner strength, resilience, and determination.

5. Enhanced Range of Motion: The extended leg in this pose provides a gentle stretch to the hamstrings and calf muscles, improving flexibility.

Variations and Adaptations

Chair Yoga celebrates adaptability, and Seated Warrior II offers several variations to suit your individual needs:

1. Supported Seated Warrior II: If balance is a concern, you can hold onto the sides of your chair for added stability.

2. Half Seated Warrior II: For a more accessible variation, practice the pose with one foot extended forward while the other remains grounded.

3. Dynamic Seated Warrior II: Incorporate dynamic movements by transitioning in and out of the pose with your breath, enhancing the flow and strength-building aspect of the practice.

4. Warrior II with Breath Emphasis: Focus on deep, intentional breaths to connect with the inner warrior, allowing your breath to guide you through the practice.

Closing Thoughts

Seated Warrior II in Chair Yoga is an embodiment of the powerful synergy between strength and grace. It teaches you that power doesn't always require force; it can be harnessed through balance and poise. Through this practice, you nurture the physical health of your body while connecting with your inner warrior, resolute and poised, ready to face life's challenges with grace. Let Seated Warrior II be your guide to unlocking your inner power, cultivating resilience, and embracing the grace that comes from within. In the dynamic stance of your body, you'll discover the profound dance of strength and elegance that Chair Yoga offers. May your journey be guided by the warrior's spirit within, inspiring you to face each day with courage, grace, and an unwavering sense of power.

CHAPTER 7
Seated Tree Pose

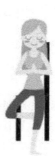

Seated Tree Pose, an embodiment of grace and balance within Chair Yoga, takes center stage in this chapter. We'll delve into the art of Seated Tree Pose, uncovering its multifaceted benefits, versatile adaptations, and the profound sense of rooted elegance and balance it can bring to your practice. In this pose, you'll discover that even while seated, you can find the calm strength of a tree.

The Seated Tree Pose Unveiled

Seated Tree Pose, inspired by its traditional standing counterpart, invites you to cultivate poise and equilibrium while seated comfortably in a chair. This pose beautifully symbolizes the rooted elegance of a tree, finding both balance and grace within.

To practice Seated Tree Pose in a chair:

1. Begin by sitting tall in your chair, with your feet flat on the ground and hip-width apart.

2. Place your hands on your thighs, palms facing downward, or rest them on your lap with palms facing upward.

3. Inhale deeply, elongating your spine, and exhale slowly, relaxing your shoulders.

4. On an inhale, extend one leg forward, keeping the foot flat on the ground.

5. As you exhale, bring the sole of your opposite foot to your inner thigh, resting it gently and creating a "V" shape with your legs.

6. Ensure your raised foot is above or below the knee, avoiding direct pressure on the joint.

7. Find your balance in this position, maintaining a strong and steady gaze forward.

8. If comfortable, bring your hands to your heart center in a prayer position, or simply rest them on your lap.

9. Hold this posture for several breaths, feeling the rooted elegance and inner balance it invokes.

10. To release, exhale and lower your raised foot to the ground, returning to the starting position.

11. Repeat the pose on the other side, maintaining balance between both sides of your body.

The Benefits of Seated Tree Pose

1. Balance and Alignment: Seated Tree Pose encourages balance and alignment within the body, enhancing posture and coordination.

2. Focused Awareness: The need for concentration in this pose promotes mental clarity and mindfulness.

3. Lower Body Strength: It strengthens the muscles in the legs, especially those that support the pelvis and spine.

4. Stress Reduction: The gentle stretch and centered awareness found in this pose can help reduce stress and induce a sense of calm.

5. Cultivation of Patience: Practicing Seated Tree Pose nurtures patience as you seek balance and stability within.

Variations and Adaptations

Chair Yoga is celebrated for its adaptability, and Seated Tree Pose offers a range of variations to cater to your unique needs:

1. Supported Seated Tree Pose: Hold onto the sides of your chair or a nearby surface for added stability, especially if balance is a concern.

2. Foot Placement: Experiment with different placements for your raised foot—above or below the knee—to find what is most comfortable and balanced for you.

3. Dynamic Seated Tree Pose: Incorporate dynamic movements by gently swaying your raised leg side to side, enhancing balance and stability.

4. Tree with Arms: Lift your arms overhead and mimic the branches of a tree, reaching out and upwards to enhance the full expression of this pose.

Closing Thoughts

Seated Tree Pose in Chair Yoga serves as a reminder that even in stillness, you can embody the elegance and balance of a tree. It encourages you to find your roots deep within while reaching for the sky with grace and poise. Through this practice, you nurture both the physical health of your body and the inner grace of your spirit, fostering a sense of grounded elegance and balance in your life. Let Seated Tree Pose be your guide to rooted elegance, inner equilibrium, and the strength that comes from a profound sense of balance. In the poised stance of your body, you'll discover the profound dance of strength and grace that Chair Yoga offers. May your journey be guided by the wisdom of the trees, inspiring you to find balance, serenity, and the quiet strength of a seated tree in all aspects of your life.

CHAPTER 8
Seated Pigeon Pose

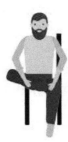

Seated Pigeon Pose, a gentle yet profound posture in Chair Yoga, takes center stage in this chapter. We'll explore the art of Seated Pigeon Pose, uncovering its myriad benefits, versatile adaptations, and the profound sense of release, flexibility, and inner harmony it can bring to your practice. This pose allows you to dive deep into your body and find freedom even while seated.

The Seated Pigeon Pose Unveiled

Seated Pigeon Pose, adapted from its traditional variation, offers an accessible way to open up the hips, relieve tension, and enhance flexibility while seated in a chair. This pose gracefully combines the elements of poise and surrender.

To practice Seated Pigeon Pose in a chair:

1. Begin by sitting tall in your chair, with your feet flat on the ground and hip-width apart.

2. Place your hands on your thighs, palms facing downward, or rest them on your lap with palms facing upward.

3. Inhale deeply, elongating your spine, and exhale slowly, relaxing your shoulders.

4. On an inhale, lift one foot off the ground and cross your ankle over the opposite thigh, creating a figure-four shape with your legs.

5. Flex the raised foot to protect your knee joint, and make sure your raised knee is pointing away from your body.

6. Gently press the raised knee downward, creating a stretch in the hip area.

7. Find your balance in this position, maintaining a strong and steady gaze forward.

8. If comfortable, you can gently press your hand on the raised knee, applying a little extra pressure to deepen the stretch.

9. Hold this posture for several breaths, allowing your hips to open and any tension to dissipate.

10. To release, exhale and lower your raised foot to the ground, returning to the starting position.

11. Repeat the pose on the other side, ensuring balance between both sides of your body.

The Benefits of Seated Pigeon Pose

1. Hip Flexibility: Seated Pigeon Pose gently opens up the hips, promoting flexibility and mobility.

2. Hip Tension Release: This pose can help alleviate tension and discomfort in the hip and lower back areas, making it particularly beneficial for individuals who sit for long periods.

3. Mental Calm: The stretch in the hip area encourages relaxation and can have a calming effect on the mind.

4. Improved Posture: By opening up the hips and reducing tension, Seated Pigeon Pose can contribute to better overall posture.

5. Lower Body Awareness: This pose fosters a deeper connection with your lower body, enhancing awareness and body-mind connection.

Variations and Adaptations

Chair Yoga offers flexibility and adaptability, and Seated Pigeon Pose comes with variations to cater to your unique needs:

1. Supported Seated Pigeon: If you have balance concerns or need extra support, hold onto the sides of your chair or a nearby surface.

2. Foot Placement: Experiment with the angle at which you place your raised foot on the thigh to find the most comfortable and effective stretch.

3. Dynamic Seated Pigeon: Incorporate dynamic movements by gently rocking your raised knee side to side, allowing the hip to open gradually.

4. Pigeon with Forward Fold: Add a forward fold by hinging at the hips and leaning your torso forward over your raised leg, intensifying the stretch.

Closing Thoughts

Seated Pigeon Pose in Chair Yoga serves as a gentle yet potent gateway to release, flexibility, and inner harmony. It invites you to embrace both the strength and the surrender within your practice. Through this pose, you nurture the physical health of your body while also fostering inner calm and emotional release. Let Seated Pigeon Pose be your guide to deep release, flexibility, and the profound sense of surrender that can be found even while seated. In the poise of your body, you'll discover the profound dance of release and flexibility that Chair Yoga offers. May your journey be guided by the gentle opening of your hips, inspiring you to find freedom, balance, and inner harmony within yourself.

CHAPTER 9
Seated Leg Extension

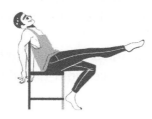

Seated Leg Extension stands as a cornerstone of Chair Yoga, offering a powerful practice that nurtures your strength, vitality, and overall well-being. In this chapter, we will dive deep into the art of Seated Leg Extension, exploring its numerous benefits, adaptable variations, and the profound sense of physical and mental empowerment it can bring to your practice. This pose, often regarded as simple, holds the potential to invigorate your entire being.

The Seated Leg Extension Unveiled

Seated Leg Extension is a foundational pose in Chair Yoga, and it's both accessible and versatile. This pose focuses on strengthening the lower body, particularly the quadriceps, and is ideal for building vitality, stability, and muscular endurance.

To practice Seated Leg Extension in a chair:

1. Begin by sitting tall in your chair, with your feet flat on the ground and hip-width apart.

2. Place your hands on your thighs, palms facing downward, or rest them on your lap with palms facing upward.

3. Inhale deeply, elongating your spine, and exhale slowly, relaxing your shoulders.

4. On an inhale, lift one leg straight out in front of you, keeping it parallel to the ground.

5. Engage your quadriceps (the muscles on the front of your thigh) to maintain the lifted leg's position.

6. Keep your toes flexed, pointing toward the ceiling, and your foot active.

7. Hold the lifted leg in place for several breaths, feeling the strength and vitality it generates.

8. To release, exhale and lower the lifted leg to the ground, returning to the starting position.

9. Repeat the pose on the other side, ensuring balance between both sides of your body.

The Benefits of Seated Leg Extension

1. Lower Body Strength: Seated Leg Extension effectively targets the quadriceps, promoting lower body strength, stability, and muscular endurance.

2. Improved Posture: Engaging your core and maintaining proper alignment in this pose can contribute to better overall posture.

3. Enhanced Circulation: Lifting your leg actively can improve blood circulation in the lower extremities, reducing the risk of blood clots and promoting vitality.

4. Mental Focus: Concentrating on maintaining the lifted leg cultivates mental clarity and mindfulness.

5. Empowerment: Seated Leg Extension can empower you by showcasing the strength and vitality within your body.

Variations and Adaptations

Chair Yoga celebrates adaptability, and Seated Leg Extension offers several variations to cater to your unique needs:

1. Supported Seated Leg Extension: Hold onto the sides of your chair or a nearby surface for added stability, especially if balance is a concern.

2. Alternate Leg Lifts: Instead of holding each leg extended for several breaths, you can alternate lifting one leg and then the other in a dynamic fashion.

3. Dynamic Seated Leg Extension: Incorporate dynamic movements by lifting and lowering your leg repeatedly with your breath, adding a flowing element to the practice.

4. Leg Extension with Ankle Weights: For those seeking more challenge, consider using ankle weights to intensify the workout.

Closing Thoughts

Seated Leg Extension in Chair Yoga offers a simple yet potent gateway to strength, vitality, and empowerment. It reminds you that strength is not limited to the gym but can be harnessed wherever you are, even while seated. Through this practice, you nurture the physical health of your body and the sense of empowerment that arises from within. Let Seated Leg Extension be your guide to cultivating strength, vitality, and a profound sense of empowerment in your life. In the poise of your lifted leg, you'll discover the profound dance of strength and vitality that Chair Yoga offers. May your journey be guided by the simple yet transformative practice of Seated Leg Extension, inspiring you to embrace your inner strength and vitality in all aspects of your life.

CHAPTER 10
Seated Cobra Pose

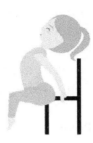

Seated Cobra Pose, a graceful and revitalizing posture in Chair Yoga, takes center stage in this chapter. We'll explore the art of Seated Cobra Pose, uncovering its multifaceted benefits, versatile adaptations, and the profound sense of vitality, flexibility, and inner grace it can bring to your practice. This pose is an invitation to embrace the awakening of your body's innate vitality and grace, all while seated in a chair.

The Seated Cobra Pose Unveiled

Seated Cobra Pose is a chair adaptation of the traditional Cobra Pose found in yoga. It encourages gentle backbending and stretching, offering an accessible way to awaken and rejuvenate the spine and surrounding muscles.

To practice Seated Cobra Pose in a chair:

1. Begin by sitting tall in your chair, with your feet flat on the ground and hip-width apart.

2. Place your hands on your thighs, palms facing downward, or rest them on your lap with palms facing upward.

3. Inhale deeply, elongating your spine, and exhale slowly, relaxing your shoulders.

4. On an inhale, engage your core muscles and gently arch your back, lifting your chest and heart upward.

5. Allow your shoulders to relax down and back, broadening across your chest.

6. Keep your gaze forward, looking straight ahead, and ensure your neck remains in a comfortable, neutral position.

7. Hold this posture for several breaths, feeling the gentle stretch along the front of your torso and the awakening of your spine.

8. To release, exhale and slowly return to an upright position, allowing your spine to come back to its neutral alignment.

The Benefits of Seated Cobra Pose

1. Spinal Flexibility: Seated Cobra Pose gently stretches and rejuvenates the spine, promoting flexibility and mitigating stiffness.

2. Improved Posture: By opening up the chest and heart center, this pose encourages an upright and confident posture.

3. Vitality and Energy: Seated Cobra Pose can boost your energy levels, providing a sense of revitalization and awakening.

4. Stress Reduction: The heart-opening aspect of this pose can help reduce stress and promote emotional well-being.

5. Respiratory Health: The expansion of the chest can enhance lung capacity and promote better breathing.

Variations and Adaptations

Chair Yoga is celebrated for its adaptability, and Seated Cobra Pose offers variations to cater to your unique needs:

1. Supported Seated Cobra: Hold onto the sides of your chair or place your hands on the armrests for added support, especially if you have balance concerns.

2. Dynamic Seated Cobra: Incorporate dynamic movements by flowing in and out of the pose with your breath, enhancing flexibility and vitality.

3. Extended Seated Cobra: Combine Seated Cobra Pose with a gentle forward fold. Inhale to lift your chest and exhale to hinge at your hips, reaching your hands toward the floor.

4. Cobra with Breath Emphasis: Focus on deep, intentional breaths to enhance the opening of the heart center and embrace the vitality it brings.

Closing Thoughts

Seated Cobra Pose in Chair Yoga serves as a gentle yet potent gateway to vitality, flexibility, and inner grace. It invites you to embrace the awakening of your body's innate vitality, all while nurturing a sense of grace and openness. Through this practice, you nurture the physical health of your body and the sense of vitality and grace that emerges from within. Let Seated Cobra Pose be your guide to embracing the vitality, flexibility, and inner grace that can be found within your own being. In the arch of your back and the opening of your heart, you'll discover the profound dance of vitality and grace that Chair Yoga offers. May your journey be guided by the awakening of your body's innate vitality, inspiring you to move through life with flexibility, grace, and a heart full of vitality.

CHAPTER 11
Seated Shoulder Stretch

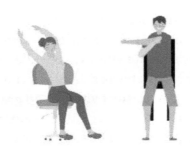

Seated Shoulder Stretch, a posture of liberation and comfort in Chair Yoga, assumes the spotlight in this chapter. We will embark on a journey to explore the art of Seated Shoulder Stretch, revealing its diverse benefits, adaptable variations, and the profound sense of freedom, ease, and relaxation it can infuse into your practice. This pose, often perceived as simple, harbors the potential to release tension and invite tranquility while seated.

The Seated Shoulder Stretch Unveiled

Seated Shoulder Stretch is a foundational pose in Chair Yoga, known for its simplicity yet profound impact on releasing tension in the upper body, particularly the shoulders, neck, and upper back. It offers a gentle way to counteract the effects of modern life, where we often find ourselves hunched over screens and desks.

To practice Seated Shoulder Stretch in a chair:

1. Begin by sitting tall in your chair, with your feet flat on the ground and hip-width apart.

2. Place your hands on your thighs, palms facing downward, or rest them on your lap with palms facing upward.

3. Inhale deeply, elongating your spine, and exhale slowly, relaxing your shoulders.

4. On an inhale, lift your right arm straight up toward the ceiling, extending it fully.

5. Exhale and gently bend your right elbow, bringing your right hand to reach down your upper back. Your fingers should be pointing downward, and your hand should be positioned between your shoulder blades.

6. Inhale, raising your left hand to the ceiling, and exhale as you bend your left elbow, bringing your left hand down your upper back. Your left hand should reach toward your right hand, and both should meet if possible.

7. If your hands do not touch, you can use a yoga strap, towel, or belt to bridge the gap between your hands, gently holding onto both ends.

8. Once your hands are connected or secured by a prop, breathe deeply and expand your chest, gently arching your back and opening your heart.

9. Hold this posture for several breaths, allowing your shoulders and chest to gently stretch and release tension.

10. To release, gently unravel your hands or release the strap, and return to an upright seated position.

11. Repeat the stretch on the other side, ensuring balance between both sides of your body.

The Benefits of Seated Shoulder Stretch

1. Shoulder and Neck Relief: Seated Shoulder Stretch effectively targets tension in the shoulders and neck, offering relief from discomfort and stiffness.

2. Chest Opening: This pose encourages the opening of the chest and heart center, enhancing posture and reducing the effects of hunching.

3. Stress Reduction: The release of tension in the upper body can alleviate stress and promote emotional well-being.

4. Improved Respiratory Function: By expanding the chest, this stretch can enhance lung capacity and improve breathing.

5. Increased Blood Flow: Seated Shoulder Stretch can stimulate blood circulation in the upper body, promoting vitality and relaxation.

Variations and Adaptations

Chair Yoga is celebrated for its adaptability, and Seated Shoulder Stretch offers variations to cater to your unique needs:

1. Supported Seated Shoulder Stretch: Hold onto the sides of your chair or a nearby surface with your free hand for added support, especially if you have balance concerns.

2. Gentle Shoulder Stretch: If reaching both hands behind your back is challenging, simply focus on reaching one hand down your upper back while keeping the other hand on your lap.

3. Dynamic Shoulder Stretch: Incorporate dynamic movements by gently pulsing your hands up and down your back with your breath, enhancing the release of tension.

4. Shoulder Stretch with Breath Emphasis: Focus on deep, intentional breaths to enhance the expansion of the chest and the sense of release and ease.

Closing Thoughts

Seated Shoulder Stretch in Chair Yoga serves as a reminder that simplicity can hold great power. It invites you to release tension and embrace ease and freedom within your body, all while seated in a chair. Through this practice, you nurture the physical health of your upper body and the sense of relaxation and ease that arises from within. Let Seated Shoulder Stretch be your guide to releasing tension, embracing freedom, and finding tranquility within your own being. In the reach of your hands and the expansion of your chest, you'll discover the profound dance of freedom and ease that Chair Yoga offers. May your journey be guided by the simple yet transformative practice of Seated Shoulder Stretch, inspiring you to move through life with relaxation, freedom, and a heart full of ease.

CHAPTER 12
Seated Neck Rolls

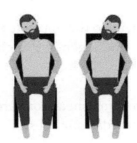

Seated Neck Rolls, a gentle yet profoundly liberating practice in Chair Yoga, takes center stage in this chapter. We'll embark on a journey to explore the art of Seated Neck Rolls, unveiling its numerous benefits, adaptable variations, and the profound sense of relaxation, mobility, and inner peace it can bring to your practice. This deceptively simple practice holds the potential to release tension and foster tranquility while seated.

The Seated Neck Rolls Unveiled

Seated Neck Rolls are a foundational practice in Chair Yoga, offering a gentle way to release tension and increase mobility in the neck and shoulders. They provide a moment of respite in our often busy lives, allowing us to reconnect with our bodies and find peace within.

To practice Seated Neck Rolls in a chair:

1. Begin by sitting tall in your chair, with your feet flat on the ground and hip-width apart.

2. Place your hands on your thighs, palms facing downward, or rest them on your lap with palms facing upward.

3. Inhale deeply, elongating your spine, and exhale slowly, relaxing your shoulders.

4. On an inhale, gently lower your chin towards your chest, feeling a gentle stretch along the back of your neck.

5. As you exhale, slowly roll your head to one side, bringing your right ear towards your right shoulder. Feel a gentle stretch along the left side of your neck.

6. Inhale and continue to roll your head gently back, allowing your gaze to drift towards the ceiling.

7. Exhale as you roll your head to the opposite side, bringing your left ear towards your left shoulder. Feel a gentle stretch along the right side of your neck.

8. Inhale and continue to roll your head forward, completing the circle and returning your chin towards your chest.

9. Repeat this gentle rolling motion for several rounds, moving at your own pace and paying attention to any areas of tension or restriction.

10. After a few rounds in one direction, switch to the other direction, ensuring balance and mobility in both directions.

11. To conclude, return your head to a neutral position, with your chin parallel to the ground.

The Benefits of Seated Neck Rolls

1. Neck Mobility: Seated Neck Rolls gently increase the range of motion in the neck, helping to alleviate stiffness and tension.

2. Stress Reduction: The slow, mindful movements of this practice can reduce stress and promote a sense of relaxation and tranquility.

3. Improved Posture: By releasing tension in the neck and shoulders, Seated Neck Rolls contribute to better overall posture.

4. Mind-Body Connection: Practicing mindful movement fosters a deeper connection between your body and mind, enhancing body awareness.

5. Mental Clarity: The focus on the breath and movement in this practice can lead to mental clarity and a sense of inner peace.

Variations and Adaptations

Chair Yoga thrives on adaptability, and Seated Neck Rolls offer variations to cater to your unique needs:

1. Supported Seated Neck Rolls: If you have balance concerns or need added support, you can hold onto the sides of your chair for stability.

2. Slow and Mindful Rolls: Emphasize slow, mindful movements, pausing at any points of tension or discomfort to breathe into those areas.

3. Neck Rolls with Breath Emphasis: Sync your breath with the movement, inhaling as you roll your head in one direction and exhaling as you roll in the other direction.

4. Extended Neck Rolls: Extend the rolling motion to include the shoulders, gently rolling them forward and backward as you move your head.

Closing Thoughts

Seated Neck Rolls in Chair Yoga serve as a gentle yet powerful gateway to relaxation, mobility, and inner peace. They invite you to release tension and foster tranquility within your body and mind, all while seated in a chair. Through this practice, you nurture the physical health of your neck and shoulders and the sense of relaxation and inner peace that emerges from within. Let Seated Neck Rolls be your guide to unlocking relaxation, mobility, and a profound sense of peace in your life. In the circular motion of your head, you'll discover the profound dance of relaxation and mobility that Chair Yoga offers. May your journey be guided by the simple yet transformative practice of Seated Neck Rolls, inspiring you to move through life with relaxation, mobility, and a heart full of inner peace.

CHAPTER 13
Seated Ankle Rolls

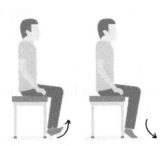

Seated Ankle Rolls, a subtle yet immensely beneficial practice in Chair Yoga, takes center stage in this chapter. We will embark on a journey to explore the art of Seated Ankle Rolls, revealing its multifaceted benefits, adaptable variations, and the profound sense of mobility, groundedness, and body awareness it can bring to your practice. This deceptively simple practice holds the power to nurture your ankles, enhance balance, and foster a sense of inner calm while seated.

The Seated Ankle Rolls Unveiled

Seated Ankle Rolls are a foundational practice in Chair Yoga, offering a gentle way to improve ankle mobility and increase body awareness. This practice is especially valuable for those who spend extended periods sitting or have limited mobility.

To practice Seated Ankle Rolls in a chair:

1. Begin by sitting tall in your chair, with your feet flat on the ground and hip-width apart.

2. Place your hands on your thighs, palms facing downward, or rest them on your lap with palms facing upward.

3. Inhale deeply, elongating your spine, and exhale slowly, relaxing your shoulders.

4. On an inhale, lift your right foot slightly off the ground, keeping your toes in contact with the floor.

5. Begin to gently rotate your right ankle in a clockwise direction, making small circles with your foot.

6. Continue the circular motion for several breaths, feeling the gentle stretch and mobility in your ankle.

7. After a few rounds in one direction, switch to counterclockwise circles to balance the movement.

8. Lower your right foot back to the ground and take a moment to observe any sensations in your ankle.

9. Repeat the practice with your left foot, lifting it slightly off the ground and making both clockwise and counterclockwise ankle circles.

10. After completing the ankle rolls on both sides, place both feet flat on the ground and take a few deep breaths to ground yourself.

The Benefits of Seated Ankle Rolls

1. Improved Ankle Mobility: Seated Ankle Rolls gently increase the range of motion in the ankles, promoting flexibility and mobility.

2. Groundedness: This practice encourages a sense of groundedness and connection with the earth through the feet.

3. Body Awareness: Seated Ankle Rolls foster body awareness by drawing your attention to the sensations in your ankles.

4. Stress Reduction: The mindful movement of this practice can reduce stress and promote relaxation.

5. Enhanced Balance: Regular practice of Seated Ankle Rolls can improve balance, which is essential for everyday activities.

Variations and Adaptations

Chair Yoga thrives on adaptability, and Seated Ankle Rolls offer variations to cater to your unique needs:

1. Supported Ankle Rolls: If you have difficulty lifting your foot off the ground or need added support, use your hands to gently guide the ankle in the circular motion.

2. Slow and Mindful Rolls: Emphasize slow, mindful movements, paying close attention to the sensations in your ankles as you roll them.

3. Ankle Rolls with Breath Emphasis: Sync your breath with the movement, inhaling as you circle your ankle in one direction and exhaling as you circle in the other direction.

4. Extended Ankle Rolls: If you're comfortable with the basic movement, extend the circles to make them larger, providing a deeper stretch.

Closing Thoughts

Seated Ankle Rolls in Chair Yoga serve as a gentle yet potent gateway to mobility, groundedness, and body awareness. They invite you to nurture your ankles and reconnect with the earth beneath you, all while seated in a chair. Through this practice, you nurture the physical health of your ankles and the sense of groundedness and body awareness that arises from within. Let Seated Ankle Rolls be your guide to nurturing mobility, groundedness, and a profound sense of presence in your life. In the circular motion of your ankles, you'll discover the profound dance of mobility and groundedness that Chair Yoga offers. May your journey be guided by the simple yet transformative practice of Seated Ankle Rolls, inspiring you to move through life with mobility, groundedness, and a heart full of presence.

CHAPTER 14
Seated Eagle Arms

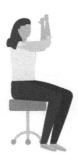

Seated Eagle Arms, an embodiment of grace and balance within Chair Yoga, takes center stage in this chapter. We'll delve into the art of Seated Eagle Arms, uncovering its multifaceted benefits, versatile adaptations, and the profound sense of grace, balance, and poise it can bring to your practice. In this pose, you'll discover that even while seated, you can find the elegance and unity of an eagle in flight.

The Seated Eagle Arms Unveiled

Seated Eagle Arms is a modified version of the traditional Eagle Pose in yoga, adapted for seated practice in a chair. It encourages you to cultivate poise, balance, and flexibility while seated comfortably.

To practice Seated Eagle Arms in a chair:

1. Begin by sitting tall in your chair, with your feet flat on the ground and hip-width apart.

2. Place your hands on your thighs, palms facing downward, or rest them on your lap with palms facing upward.

3. Inhale deeply, elongating your spine, and exhale slowly, relaxing your shoulders.

4. On an inhale, raise both arms to shoulder height, parallel to the ground, palms facing forward.

5. Exhale, and sweep your right arm under your left arm, crossing at the elbows. Your right elbow should rest on top of your left elbow, and your forearms should be perpendicular to the ground, creating an "X" shape with your arms.

6. If possible, bring your palms together, pressing them gently. If your palms don't reach, you can touch the back of your hands or simply hold onto opposite shoulders.

7. Engage your core and maintain a steady gaze forward.

8. Hold this posture for several breaths, feeling the graceful intertwining of your arms and the sense of unity and balance it invokes.

9. To release, inhale and open your arms wide, returning to the starting position.

10. Repeat the pose, this time crossing your left arm over your right, ensuring balance between both sides of your body.

The Benefits of Seated Eagle Arms

1. Shoulder and Upper Back Stretch: Seated Eagle Arms gently stretch the shoulders and upper back, releasing tension and promoting flexibility.

2. Improved Posture: By aligning and opening the shoulders, this pose contributes to better overall posture.

3. Balance and Coordination: The need for balance and coordination in this pose enhances physical and mental equilibrium.

4. Focused Awareness: Concentrating on the intertwining of your arms fosters mindfulness and inner balance.

5. Stress Reduction: The deliberate and focused nature of this practice can help reduce stress and promote a sense of inner calm.

Variations and Adaptations

Chair Yoga is celebrated for its adaptability, and Seated Eagle Arms offers variations to cater to your unique needs:

1. Supported Seated Eagle Arms: If you have balance concerns or need extra support, hold onto the sides of your chair or a nearby surface for added stability.

2. Dynamic Seated Eagle Arms: Incorporate dynamic movements by gently opening and closing your crossed arms with your breath, enhancing the stretch and flexibility.

3. Eagle Arms with a Forward Fold: Combine Seated Eagle Arms with a forward fold by hinging at the hips and leaning your torso forward over your thighs, intensifying the stretch and promoting relaxation.

4. Extended Seated Eagle Arms: Extend your arms away from your body, keeping them parallel to the ground, to intensify the stretch and engage more muscles in your upper body.

Closing Thoughts

Seated Eagle Arms in Chair Yoga serves as a reminder that even in stillness, you can embody the grace and balance of an eagle in flight. It encourages you to find unity and balance within yourself while seated comfortably. Through this practice, you nurture the physical health of your upper body and the inner grace and poise that arise from within. Let Seated Eagle Arms be your guide to embracing grace, balance, and unity in your life. In the intertwining of your arms and the unity they create, you'll discover the profound dance of grace and balance that Chair Yoga offers. May your journey be guided by the elegance and unity of Seated Eagle Arms, inspiring you to find poise, balance, and a heart full of grace in all aspects of your life.

CHAPTER 15
Seated Garland Pose

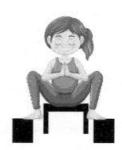

Seated Garland Pose, a practice of flexibility and groundedness within Chair Yoga, takes center stage in this chapter. We will dive deep into the art of Seated Garland Pose, unveiling its numerous benefits, adaptable variations, and the profound sense of flexibility, stability, and inner grounding it can bring to your practice. In this pose, you'll discover how even in a chair, you can embody the openness and rootedness of a garland.

The Seated Garland Pose Unveiled

Seated Garland Pose, adapted from its traditional variation, offers an accessible way to embrace flexibility and groundedness while seated in a chair. This pose gracefully combines the elements of flexibility and stability, inviting you to find your center.

To practice Seated Garland Pose in a chair:

1. Begin by sitting tall in your chair, with your feet flat on the ground and hip-width apart.

2. Place your hands on your thighs, palms facing downward, or rest them on your lap with palms facing upward.

3. Inhale deeply, elongating your spine, and exhale slowly, relaxing your shoulders.

4. On an inhale, slide your feet apart, widening your stance to the edges of the chair.

5. Exhale, and angle your feet outward at approximately 45 degrees, allowing your knees to gently open.

6. Inhale and lift your chest, maintaining an upright and elongated spine.

7. Exhale and engage your core as you gently press your elbows against your inner thighs, encouraging your knees to open wider.

8. If comfortable, you can bring your palms together in a prayer position, pressing your hands firmly together to deepen the stretch.

9. Hold this posture for several breaths, feeling the gentle opening of your hips and the sense of stability and grounding.

10. To release, exhale and lower your hands to your thighs or lap, then gently bring your feet back to hip-width apart.

The Benefits of Seated Garland Pose

1. Hip Flexibility: Seated Garland Pose gently opens up the hips, promoting flexibility and mobility.

2. Lower Back Relief: This pose can help alleviate tension and discomfort in the lower back, making it beneficial for individuals who sit for extended periods.

3. Stability and Grounding: Seated Garland Pose fosters a sense of stability and grounding, promoting a feeling of security and centeredness.

4. Improved Posture: By opening up the hips and maintaining an upright spine, this pose contributes to better overall posture.

5. Mind-Body Connection: Practicing this pose enhances body awareness and the connection between your physical and mental states.

Variations and Adaptations

Chair Yoga celebrates adaptability, and Seated Garland Pose offers variations to cater to your unique needs:

1. Supported Seated Garland: Hold onto the sides of your chair or place your hands on a nearby surface for added support, especially if balance is a concern.

2. Dynamic Seated Garland: Incorporate dynamic movements by gently rocking your pelvis side to side, allowing the hips to open gradually.

3. Garland with Forward Fold: Add a forward fold by hinging at the hips and leaning your torso forward over your thighs, intensifying the stretch.

4. Garland with Ankle Weights: For those seeking a greater challenge, consider using ankle weights to enhance the workout.

Closing Thoughts

Seated Garland Pose in Chair Yoga serves as a gentle yet potent gateway to flexibility, stability, and inner grounding. It invites you to find your center and embrace the flexibility that exists within you, even while seated. Through this practice, you nurture the physical health of your body and the sense of stability and grounding that emerges from within. Let Seated Garland Pose be your guide to embodying flexibility, stability, and a profound sense of grounding in your life. In the openness of your hips and the rootedness of your stance, you'll discover the profound dance of flexibility and groundedness that Chair Yoga offers. May your journey be guided by the graceful and grounded energy of Seated Garland Pose, inspiring you to find flexibility, stability, and a heart full of groundedness in all aspects of your life.

CHAPTER 16
Seated Side Stretch

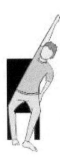

Seated Side Stretch, a practice of expansive movement and revitalization within Chair Yoga, takes center stage in this chapter. We'll embark on a journey to explore the art of Seated Side Stretch, revealing its numerous benefits, adaptable variations, and the profound sense of expansion, vitality, and rejuvenation it can bring to your practice. In this pose, you'll discover that even while seated, you can touch the sky and breathe new life into your being.

The Seated Side Stretch Unveiled

Seated Side Stretch is a modified version of traditional side stretches in yoga, adapted for seated practice in a chair. This pose encourages you to embrace expansive movement and revitalize your body, even while seated comfortably.

To practice Seated Side Stretch in a chair:

1. Begin by sitting tall in your chair, with your feet flat on the ground and hip-width apart.

2. Place your hands on your thighs, palms facing downward, or rest them on your lap with palms facing upward.

3. Inhale deeply, elongating your spine, and exhale slowly, relaxing your shoulders.

4. On an inhale, raise both arms overhead, extending them fully toward the ceiling, palms facing each other.

5. Exhale and engage your core muscles, grounding your sit bones into the chair.

6. Inhale once more, lengthening through your spine, and exhale as you lean gently to one side, creating a crescent shape with your upper body.

7. Keep both feet flat on the ground, ensuring stability.

8. Continue to breathe deeply as you feel the stretch along the side of your body, from your fingertips down to your hips.

9. Hold this posture for several breaths, maintaining the stretch and feeling a sense of expansion and vitality.

10. To release, inhale and return to an upright position, then exhale as you lean to the opposite side, repeating the stretch on the other side.

11. Ensure balance between both sides of your body by holding the stretch for an equal amount of time on each side.

The Benefits of Seated Side Stretch

1. Spinal Flexibility: Seated Side Stretch encourages flexibility in the spine, alleviating stiffness and enhancing mobility.

2. Improved Posture: By expanding the side body, this pose contributes to better overall posture.

3. Vitality and Energy: The expansive nature of this pose can boost your energy levels, providing a sense of revitalization and renewal.

4. Stress Reduction: The stretching and deep breathing involved in this practice can help reduce stress and promote emotional well-being.

5. Enhanced Lung Capacity: By creating space in the side body, Seated Side Stretch can enhance lung capacity and improve breathing.

Variations and Adaptations

Chair Yoga is celebrated for its adaptability, and Seated Side Stretch offers variations to cater to your unique needs:

1. Supported Seated Side Stretch: Hold onto the sides of your chair or place one hand on the chair and the other on your hip for added support, especially if you have balance concerns.

2. Dynamic Seated Side Stretch: Incorporate dynamic movements by gently pulsing up and down in the stretch with your breath, deepening the sensation of expansion.

3. Seated Side Stretch with Arm Variation: As you lean to one side, extend your top arm over your head, creating an even greater stretch along the side body.

4. Extended Seated Side Stretch: For a more intense stretch, lean farther to the side, reaching your hand closer to the ground while maintaining stability.

Closing Thoughts

Seated Side Stretch in Chair Yoga serves as a gentle yet potent gateway to expansion, vitality, and rejuvenation. It invites you to embrace the expansive movement and revitalize your body, even while seated. Through this practice, you nurture the physical health of your spine and the sense of expansion and vitality that arises from within. Let Seated Side Stretch be your guide to expanding your horizons, cultivating vitality, and rejuvenating your being. In the stretch of your side body and the upward reach of your arms, you'll discover the profound dance of expansion and vitality that Chair Yoga offers. May your journey be guided by the expansive and revitalizing energy of Seated Side Stretch, inspiring you to reach for the sky and breathe new life into all aspects of your existence.

CHAPTER 17
Seated Warrior III

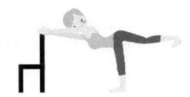

Seated Warrior III, a practice of strength, balance, and poise within Chair Yoga, takes center stage in this chapter. We'll embark on a journey to explore the art of Seated Warrior III, unveiling its numerous benefits, adaptable variations, and the profound sense of strength, stability, and inner poise it can bring to your practice. In this pose, you'll discover that even while seated, you can embody the grace and power of a warrior.

The Seated Warrior III Unveiled

Seated Warrior III is a modified version of the traditional Warrior III Pose in yoga, adapted for seated practice in a chair. This pose encourages you to find balance, strength, and poise while seated comfortably.

To practice Seated Warrior III in a chair:

1. Begin by sitting tall in your chair, with your feet flat on the ground and hip-width apart.

2. Place your hands on your thighs, palms facing downward, or rest them on your lap with palms facing upward.

3. Inhale deeply, elongating your spine, and exhale slowly, relaxing your shoulders.

4. On an inhale, engage your core muscles and lift your right foot off the ground, extending it straight out in front of you.

5. Flex your right foot, pointing your toes toward the ceiling.

6. As you exhale, begin to lean forward slightly from your hips, keeping your back straight and your chest lifted.

7. Simultaneously, reach your arms forward and parallel to the ground, palms facing each other.

8. Continue to breathe deeply as you feel the engagement in your core and the strength in your extended leg.

9. Hold this posture for several breaths, maintaining your balance and feeling a sense of strength and poise.

10. To release, inhale and return your extended foot to the ground, then exhale as you return to an upright seated position.

11. Repeat the pose on the other side, lifting and extending your left foot.

The Benefits of Seated Warrior III

1. Leg Strength: Seated Warrior III engages and strengthens the leg muscles, particularly the quadriceps, hamstrings, and calf muscles.

2. Core Stability: The pose challenges the core muscles, promoting stability and strength in the abdominal and lower back muscles.

3. Improved Posture: By encouraging a straight back and lifted chest, this pose contributes to better overall posture.

4. Balance and Coordination: Seated Warrior III enhances balance and coordination, both physically and mentally.

5. Mind-Body Connection: Practicing this pose fosters a deeper connection between your body and mind, enhancing body awareness.

Variations and Adaptations

Chair Yoga thrives on adaptability, and Seated Warrior III offers variations to cater to your unique needs:

1. Supported Seated Warrior III: Hold onto the sides of your chair or place your hands on a nearby surface for added support, especially if you have balance concerns.

2. Dynamic Seated Warrior III: Incorporate dynamic movements by lifting and lowering your extended leg and arms with your breath, enhancing the challenge and strength-building aspects.

3. Seated Warrior III with Bent Knee: If extending the leg fully is challenging, consider bending your knee slightly while maintaining the balance and poise of the pose.

4. Seated Warrior III with Leg Variation: Instead of extending your leg straight out in front, you can experiment with different leg positions, such as crossing one ankle over the other or opening your leg to the side.

Closing Thoughts

Seated Warrior III in Chair Yoga serves as a reminder that even while seated, you can embody the strength, balance, and poise of a warrior. It invites you to find your inner strength and balance while seated comfortably. Through this practice, you nurture the physical health of your legs and core muscles and the sense of strength and poise that arises from within. Let Seated Warrior III be your guide to balancing strength, stability, and inner poise in your life. In the extension of your leg and the reach of your arms, you'll discover the profound dance of strength and poise that Chair Yoga offers. May your journey be guided by the graceful and powerful energy of Seated Warrior III, inspiring you to find strength, stability, and a heart full of poise in all aspects of your life.

CHAPTER 18

Seated Boat Pose

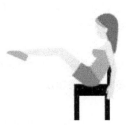

Seated Boat Pose, a practice of core strength and balance within Chair Yoga, takes center stage in this chapter. We will embark on a journey to explore the art of Seated Boat Pose, unveiling its numerous benefits, adaptable variations, and the profound sense of core strength, balance, and inner stability it can bring to your practice. In this pose, you'll discover that even while seated, you can sail through the waters of strength and stability.

The Seated Boat Pose Unveiled

Seated Boat Pose is a modified version of the traditional Boat Pose in yoga, adapted for seated practice in a chair. This pose invites you to engage your core muscles and find balance and strength while seated comfortably.

To practice Seated Boat Pose in a chair:

1. Begin by sitting tall in your chair, with your feet flat on the ground and hip-width apart.

2. Place your hands on your thighs, palms facing downward, or rest them on your lap with palms facing upward.

3. Inhale deeply, elongating your spine, and exhale slowly, relaxing your shoulders.

4. On an inhale, engage your core muscles and lift both feet off the ground, bringing your knees toward your chest.

5. Extend your arms forward, parallel to the ground, palms facing each other.

6. Balance on your sit bones and find a comfortable position where you feel stable and engaged.

7. Continue to breathe deeply as you feel the engagement in your core and the balance in your seated posture.

8. Hold this posture for several breaths, maintaining your balance and feeling a sense of core strength and stability.

9. To release, inhale and lower your feet back to the ground, then exhale as you return to an upright seated position.

The Benefits of Seated Boat Pose

1. Core Strengthening: Seated Boat Pose engages and strengthens the core muscles, including the abdominal and lower back muscles.

2. Improved Posture: By encouraging an upright and balanced seated posture, this pose contributes to better overall alignment.

3. Balance and Coordination: Seated Boat Pose enhances balance and coordination, both physically and mentally.

4. Stress Reduction: The focused and controlled nature of this practice can help reduce stress and promote emotional well-being.

5. Increased Awareness: Practicing this pose fosters a deeper awareness of the connection between your body and breath, enhancing mindfulness.

Variations and Adaptations

Chair Yoga thrives on adaptability, and Seated Boat Pose offers variations to cater to your unique needs:

1. Supported Seated Boat Pose: Hold onto the sides of your chair or place your hands on a nearby surface for added support, especially if you have balance concerns.

2. Dynamic Seated Boat Pose: Incorporate dynamic movements by gently lifting and lowering your legs with your breath, enhancing the challenge and strength-building aspects.

3. Seated Boat Pose with Knee Variation: If lifting both feet off the ground is challenging, consider keeping one foot on the ground while lifting and extending the other leg, alternating between legs.

4. Seated Boat Pose with Leg Variation: Experiment with different leg positions, such as crossing one ankle over the other or opening your legs to the sides, to add variety to your practice.

Closing Thoughts

Seated Boat Pose in Chair Yoga serves as a reminder that even while seated, you can harness the power of core strength and balance. It invites you to find your inner stability and engage your core while seated comfortably. Through this practice, you nurture the physical health of your core muscles and the sense of strength and stability that arises from within. Let Seated Boat Pose be your guide to harnessing core strength, balance, and inner stability in your life. In the engagement of your core and the balance you find, you'll discover the profound dance of strength and stability that Chair Yoga offers. May your journey be guided by the strong and steady energy of Seated Boat Pose, inspiring you to find core strength, balance, and a heart full of stability in all aspects of your life.

CHAPTER 19
Seated Extended Triangle Pose

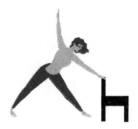

Seated Extended Triangle Pose, a practice of expansion, alignment, and mindful awareness within Chair Yoga, takes center stage in this chapter. We'll embark on a journey to explore the art of Seated Extended Triangle Pose, unveiling its numerous benefits, adaptable variations, and the profound sense of expansion, alignment, and inner awareness it can bring to your practice. In this pose, you'll discover that even while seated, you can reach for the farthest horizons of your being.

The Seated Extended Triangle Pose Unveiled

Seated Extended Triangle Pose is a modified version of the traditional Extended Triangle Pose in yoga, adapted for seated practice in a chair. This pose encourages you to find alignment, expansion, and mindfulness while seated comfortably.

To practice Seated Extended Triangle Pose in a chair:

1. Begin by sitting tall in your chair, with your feet flat on the ground and hip-width apart.

2. Place your hands on your thighs, palms facing downward, or rest them on your lap with palms facing upward.

3. Inhale deeply, elongating your spine, and exhale slowly, relaxing your shoulders.

4. On an inhale, engage your core muscles and extend your right leg out to the side, keeping your foot flexed and toes pointing forward.

5. Exhale as you reach your right arm up and overhead, extending it fully toward the left side, palm facing down.

6. Inhale and lengthen your spine, creating space between your ribs and hips.

7. Exhale and tilt your upper body to the left, maintaining the extension through your right arm.

8. Reach your left arm down toward your left knee, shin, or ankle, depending on your flexibility and comfort.

9. Turn your gaze upward, directing your attention toward your extended arm, or keep it forward for a gentler stretch.

10. Hold this posture for several breaths, feeling the stretch along the right side of your body and the sense of expansion and alignment.

11. To release, inhale and return your right arm to an upright position, then exhale as you bring your right foot back to the ground.

12. Repeat the pose on the other side, extending your left leg and reaching your left arm up and over to the right.

The Benefits of Seated Extended Triangle Pose

1. Spinal Alignment: Seated Extended Triangle Pose encourages proper spinal alignment, promoting a straight back and better posture.

2. Leg and Hip Flexibility: The pose stretches the inner thighs and hamstrings, enhancing flexibility in the legs and hips.

3. Core Engagement: Engaging the core muscles helps stabilize the posture, leading to improved core strength and stability.

4. Mindful Awareness: The focused and controlled nature of this practice cultivates mindfulness and inner awareness.

5. Improved Circulation: Stretching the sides of the body can enhance circulation and relieve tension in the upper body.

Variations and Adaptations

Chair Yoga thrives on adaptability, and Seated Extended Triangle Pose offers variations to cater to your unique needs:

1. Supported Seated Extended Triangle: Hold onto the sides of your chair or place your hands on a nearby surface for added support, especially if you have balance concerns.

2. Dynamic Seated Extended Triangle: Incorporate dynamic movements by gently pulsing up and down in the stretch with your breath, deepening the sensation of expansion and alignment.

3. Seated Extended Triangle with Arm Variation: Experiment with different arm positions, such as placing your extended arm on your lower back or reaching it behind your chair for additional opening in the chest and shoulders.

4. Seated Extended Triangle with Leg Variation: Instead of extending your leg straight out to the side, try bending your knee slightly or placing your foot on the ground for a gentler stretch.

Closing Thoughts

Seated Extended Triangle Pose in Chair Yoga serves as a reminder that even while seated, you can expand your horizons, find alignment, and cultivate mindful awareness. It invites you to reach for the farthest horizons of your being while seated comfortably. Through this practice, you nurture the physical health of your spine and the sense of expansion, alignment, and inner awareness that arises from within. Let Seated Extended Triangle Pose be your guide to expanding your horizons, finding alignment, and cultivating mindful awareness in your life. In the extension of your arm and leg, you'll discover the profound dance of expansion and alignment that Chair Yoga offers. May your journey be guided by the expansive and aligned energy of Seated Extended Triangle Pose, inspiring you to reach for the farthest horizons of your being and find a heart full of mindful awareness in all aspects of your life.

CHAPTER 20
Seated Puppy Pose

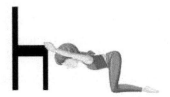

Seated Puppy Pose, a practice of surrender, release, and deep stretching within Chair Yoga, takes center stage in this chapter. We'll embark on a journey to explore the art of Seated Puppy Pose, unveiling its numerous benefits, adaptable variations, and the profound sense of surrender, release, and inner peace it can bring to your practice. In this pose, you'll discover that even while seated, you can experience the profound liberation of letting go.

The Seated Puppy Pose Unveiled

Seated Puppy Pose is a modified version of the traditional Puppy Pose in yoga, adapted for seated practice in a chair. This pose encourages you to find surrender, release, and deep stretching while seated comfortably.

To practice Seated Puppy Pose in a chair:

1. Begin by sitting tall in your chair, with your feet flat on the ground and hip-width apart.

2. Place your hands on your thighs, palms facing downward, or rest them on your lap with palms facing upward.

3. Inhale deeply, elongating your spine, and exhale slowly, relaxing your shoulders.

4. On an inhale, engage your core muscles and lift your arms overhead, extending them fully toward the ceiling, palms facing each other.

5. Exhale and hinge at your hips, folding forward with a straight back.

6. Reach your arms forward and downward, allowing them to rest on the seat of the chair between your legs.

7. Keep your head and neck aligned with your spine, avoiding any strain on your neck.

8. Continue to breathe deeply as you feel the stretch along your spine, shoulders, and the backs of your arms and legs.

9. Hold this posture for several breaths, focusing on surrendering and releasing any tension.

10. To release, inhale and slowly lift your torso back to an upright position, then exhale as you lower your arms to your sides.

The Benefits of Seated Puppy Pose

1. Spinal Release: Seated Puppy Pose encourages spinal release and stretching, promoting flexibility and relieving tension in the back.

2. Shoulder and Arm Stretch: The pose stretches the shoulders and the backs of the arms, which can be especially beneficial for those who spend extended periods sitting or working at a desk.

3. Relaxation and Stress Reduction: The surrendering nature of this practice can help release emotional and physical tension, leading to relaxation and reduced stress.

4. Hip Opening: Seated Puppy Pose provides a gentle hip opening, which can be soothing for those with tight hips.

5. Enhanced Breath Awareness: Practicing this pose fosters greater awareness of the breath and the connection between the breath and the body.

Variations and Adaptations

Chair Yoga thrives on adaptability, and Seated Puppy Pose offers variations to cater to your unique needs:

1. Supported Seated Puppy Pose: If you have difficulty reaching the chair seat or want added support, use props such as a cushion or folded blanket on the chair to rest your arms on.

2. Dynamic Seated Puppy Pose: Incorporate dynamic movements by gently swaying or rocking in the stretch with your breath, deepening the sensation of surrender and release.

3. Seated Puppy Pose with Leg Variation: Experiment with different leg positions, such as crossing one ankle over the other or opening your legs to the sides, to add variety to your practice.

4. Seated Puppy Pose with Neck Release: To further release tension in the neck and shoulders, gently nod your head "yes" and shake it "no" while in the pose.

Closing Thoughts

Seated Puppy Pose in Chair Yoga serves as a reminder that even while seated, you can experience profound surrender and release. It invites you to let go of tension, surrender to the present moment, and release any physical or emotional baggage. Through this practice, you nurture the physical health of your spine, shoulders, and arms, and the sense of surrender, release, and inner peace that arises from within. Let Seated Puppy Pose be your guide to discovering surrender, release, and profound inner peace in your life. In the stretch of your spine and arms, you'll discover the profound dance of surrender and release that Chair Yoga offers. May your journey be guided by the liberating and peaceful energy of Seated Puppy Pose, inspiring you to let go, surrender to the present moment, and find a heart full of inner peace in all aspects of your life.

We have reached the end and here I'd like to give you 20 short tips on how to achieve mastery in chair yoga.

1. Start Slow: Begin with gentle movements to warm up and avoid strain.

2. Comfort Matters: Use a sturdy chair with no wheels for stability.

3. Breathe Mindfully: Focus on your breath to stay present and calm.

4. Modify Poses: Adapt poses to your comfort level and physical abilities.

5. Regular Practice: Consistency is key; practice chair yoga regularly for best results.

6. Believe in Yourself: Trust that you can improve and grow through chair yoga.

7. Set Goals: Define achievable goals to track your progress and stay motivated.

8. Positive Affirmations: Use positive self-talk during practice for encouragement.

9. Celebrate Small Wins: Acknowledge and celebrate each improvement.

10. Visualize Success: Imagine yourself achieving your chair yoga goals.

11. Chair Cat-Cow: For spinal flexibility, practice the seated cat-cow stretch.

12. Seated Forward Bend: Relieve tension in your back by folding forward gently.

13. Chair Warrior Pose: Strengthen your legs and core with a seated warrior pose.

14. Chair Pigeon Pose: Ease hip tension with this seated variation of pigeon pose.

15. Chair Tree Pose: Work on balance and stability with the seated tree pose.

16. Mind-Body Connection: Recognize how chair yoga connects your physical and mental well-being.

17. Patience is a Virtue: Understand that progress may be slow but is still valuable.

18. Yoga is a Journey: Chair yoga is not just about physical fitness; it's a journey of self-discovery.

19. Gratitude: Cultivate gratitude for your body and its ability to practice yoga.

20. Oneness: Reflect on the unity of all beings as you practice chair yoga, promoting a sense of interconnectedness.

Remember, chair yoga is a practice that can bring physical, mental, and emotional benefits. These tips aim to help you stay motivated, safe, and connected to the deeper philosophical aspects of yoga while practicing in a chair.

Chair yoga is a transformative practice that transcends physical limitations, ignites mental resilience, and nurtures a profound connection to the self and the universe. It offers a path to holistic well-being, embracing both the tangible and the metaphysical aspects of our existence.

At its core, chair yoga embodies inclusivity. It welcomes individuals of all ages and physical abilities to embark on a journey toward health and self-discovery. The chair becomes a symbol of stability and support, a trustworthy companion on this voyage.

In the realm of the physical, chair yoga is a symphony of movement and stillness. It fosters flexibility, strength, and balance, all within the comforting embrace of a chair. The chair becomes an extension of oneself, enabling gentle stretches, soothing twists, and empowering poses. Through these postures, we not only nurture our bodies but also cultivate awareness. We learn to listen to the whispers of our muscles, the sighs of our joints, and the rhythm of our breath.

Yet, chair yoga is not confined to the realm of the physical. It is a sanctuary for the mind. As we engage in each asana (pose), we synchronize our breath with movement, harmonizing the chaotic symphony of our thoughts. This meditative dance guides us into the present moment, where past regrets and future anxieties cease to exist. It is here, in the realm of the present, that we discover our true essence.

Philosophically, chair yoga is a journey inward, a pilgrimage to the core of our being. It teaches us the profound lesson of patience, as we witness incremental progress over time. With each practice, we peel away the layers of doubt, insecurity, and self-criticism, revealing the radiant core of our authentic self.

Through chair yoga, we embrace gratitude. We are grateful for our bodies, with all their imperfections and idiosyncrasies, for they carry us through life's journey. The chair becomes a reminder that every inch of us is sacred, deserving of love and acceptance.

Ultimately, chair yoga unveils the interconnectedness of all things. As we extend our arms, we reach not just for the sky but for the cosmos. We realize that our breath, our movement, and our existence are interwoven with the universal rhythm. In this realization, we find a profound sense of oneness, a connection to all living beings and the world around us.

In conclusion, chair yoga is not merely a physical practice; it is a gateway to the soul. It invites us to explore the depths of our physical and mental capabilities, while simultaneously guiding us toward philosophical enlightenment. With each session, we inch closer to our true selves, embracing the wisdom that unfolds on this sacred journey. Through chair yoga, we discover that the path to self-discovery, resilience, and unity begins right where we are, in the loving embrace of a simple chair.

GOOD LUCK
IN EXPLORING
THE ART OF
CHAIR YOGA
:)

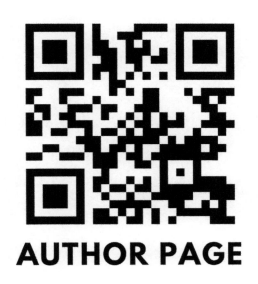

AUTHOR PAGE